Bariatric Gelatin Recipes After Surgery

A Stage-by-Stage Plan (Liquid to Regular) with Sugar-Free, Protein-First Treats

Disclaimer

This guide is provided for informational and educational purposes only and should not be interpreted as medical, nutritional, or professional advice. The author is not a licensed physician, nurse, dietitian, or mental health provider. Reading this guide does not establish a patient–provider relationship of any kind.

Always seek the guidance of a qualified healthcare professional before starting, changing, or discontinuing any supplement, diet, or lifestyle program. If you are pregnant, breastfeeding, managing a chronic medical condition, or taking prescription medications, consult your physician or pharmacist before considering any product mentioned in this guide.

The author and publisher make no representations or warranties regarding accuracy, applicability, fitness, or completeness of the information contained herein. While every effort has been made to ensure scientific accuracy and currency, medical knowledge and research evolve continually. Readers are responsible for verifying information and making decisions in consultation with licensed professionals.

Use of this guide and any information contained within it is at your own risk. The author and publisher disclaim all liability for any loss, injury, or adverse outcome that may result from the use or misuse of this material.

No supplement, diet, or practice discussed in this text is intended to diagnose, treat, cure, or prevent any disease. No outcomes or benefits are guaranteed.

Product names, supplement formulations, diet frameworks, and trademarks mentioned are the property of their respective owners and are used for identification only. Any images or illustrations that appear in related materials are licensed stock or educational placeholders.

Table of Contents

Introduction

Recovering from bariatric surgery presents unique challenges, particularly in maintaining adequate nutrition when your appetite is reduced and texture tolerance is limited. Immediately after surgery, the body's ability to handle solid foods is compromised due to reduced stomach capacity and post-operative swelling, making the choice and progression of foods critically important.

For many, the prospect of eating can feel daunting; common issues such as early satiety, food aversions, and flavor fatigue often arise. Yet, adequate protein intake remains essential to support healing, preserve lean body mass, and prevent malnutrition, especially during the rapid weight loss phase characteristic of post-surgery recovery.

Amidst these challenges, risks such as nutritional deficits, dehydration, and poor food tolerance can derail progress if dietary guidelines are not reliably followed. Skipping meals or failing to meet fluid, protein, and micronutrient targets increases the risk of complications including delayed healing, fatigue, and unpleasant symptoms like dumping syndrome or hypoglycemia.

For this reason, a thoughtfully structured, stage-wise diet plan is essential, and gelatin-based snacks present an effective and enjoyable way to bridge nutrition and satisfaction at every recovery stage.

This guide is designed specifically for adults who have undergone bariatric procedures such as gastric sleeve or gastric bypass, and are seeking practical, medically responsible guidance in using gelatin snacks to meet their nutrition goals.

You will learn to select, prepare, and enjoy sugar-free, protein-enriched gelatin treats that are tailored to your stage of recovery whether you are sipping clear liquids or transitioning to regular foods. With an emphasis on simplicity and compliance, each recipe and technique prioritizes safety, texture appropriateness, and protein density, empowering you to better adhere to medical restrictions and dietary targets.

Please note, this guide is intentionally limited in scope. It does not address non-gelatin dessert options, elaborate cooking techniques, or any use of gelatin unrelated to the needs of bariatric surgery recovery. Its purpose is not to provide individual medical or dietary prescriptions, nor does it replace direct care from your surgical or nutrition team.

Always consult your care providers before trying new recipes or products.

Throughout the chapters, you will discover:

- Clear criteria for safe food progression, from post-op clear liquids to regular textured foods, ensuring you stay within established clinical guidelines at every step.
- A curated selection of sugar-free, protein-forward gelatin snack recipes for each recovery stage, including specific advice on commercial products and homemade options that avoid unnecessary sugars or additives.
- Step-by-step preparation and safety checklists tailored to common post-bariatric concerns, like cross-contamination and careful portioning.
- Weekly meal plans and flavor variation tips to help you prevent boredom and ensure your nutritional needs are met.
- Troubleshooting guides for flavor fatigue, texture mishaps, and common digestive side effects, plus expert answers to the most frequent patient questions.
- Safe storage, batch preparation, and monitoring tools to streamline compliance and maximize safety.

As you move through the guide, practical tools including a sample seven-day gelatin snack plan will help you seamlessly incorporate gelatin-based treats into your diet, track your protein and fluid intake, and maintain momentum toward a healthier, more enjoyable post-surgery eating routine. With strategic support, you can transform gelatin snacks from a simple post-surgery staple into a creative, satisfying, and nutritionally sound part of your recovery and long-term weight management plan.

Understanding Bariatric Diet Progression and Gelatin's Role

The journey to healthy eating after bariatric surgery follows a highly structured progression through distinct dietary stages, each designed to protect the healing digestive system and maximize nutrient absorption. Immediately after surgery, eating solid foods is extremely difficult or even impossible due to reduced stomach size and post-operative swelling. To avoid regurgitation, vomiting, and complications, it is essential to move gradually from liquids to solids under clinical supervision.

This stage framework is a cornerstone of bariatric nutrition protocols and typically unfolds as follows:

1. ***Clear Liquid Stage***: This stage begins within 24 hours post-surgery. Only clear, non-carbonated, low-sugar liquids are permitted. They must be easy to digest and gentle on the healing pouch. The purpose is to ensure hydration without causing strain. Examples include water, broth, sugar-free electrolyte drinks, and clear

gelatin. Even protein-enriched clear liquids may be included if approved by your care team.

2. ***Full Liquid Stage***: After tolerating clear liquids, the next step allows more substantial fluids. These are smooth and pourable, such as meal replacement shakes, protein-fortified milks, creamy soups (strained), and gelatin snacks. At this stage, commercial or homemade gelatin that's sugar-free and potentially protein-enriched becomes a staple option, as it is soothing and provides gentle nutrition while supporting hydration.
3. ***Pureed Stage***: As healing continues, diets transition to foods pureed to a smooth consistency. Pureed proteins, soft vegetables, and fruit purees can be cautiously incorporated. Gelatin dishes can now be blended with pureed fruits or dairy, creating more varied flavors and slightly thicker textures suitable for this phase.
4. ***Soft Stage***: After successfully managing pureed foods, the introduction of soft, tender foods is allowed. This stage supports chewing and continued texture advancement, with soft-cooked eggs, canned fish, and soft gelatin parfaits or mousses adding diversity. Soft, protein-boosted gelatins and gentle add-ins are safe here, as long as portion size and tolerance are monitored.
5. ***Regular Diet***: StageThe final stage gradually reintroduces a variety of regular-texture foods,

emphasizing healthy proteins, vegetables, and whole grains in small, frequent meals. Protein-enriched gelatin desserts continue to offer convenient, structured snacking that fits the new eating lifestyle, supporting long-term weight maintenance and muscle preservation.

Progression between stages is not based strictly on time but on individual clinical criteria and dietary tolerance. Transitioning too quickly risks vomiting, nausea, and poor nutrient absorption. Before moving to the next stage, you should consistently tolerate the current stage's recommended foods without discomfort and meet minimum fluid and nutritional goals. Always consult your bariatric dietitian or surgical team before advancing through stages to ensure safe, individualized progress.

Key Nutrient Requirements After Surgery: Focus on Hydration and Protein

After bariatric surgery, the risk of malnutrition and dehydration is highest in the early recovery phases. Both hydration and protein are top priorities, as they support wound healing, minimize muscle loss, and prevent avoidable complications. However, the drastic reduction in stomach capacity often leads to a marked decrease in protein and fluid intake, especially in the first months post-surgery.

Hydration:

- Sip water and approved clear liquids throughout the day (not with meals), aiming for regular, small doses to prevent dehydration.
- Sugar-free gelatin snacks contribute to fluid intake and can be strategically rotated with other clear liquids for palatability and compliance.

Protein:

- Current bariatric guidelines recommend a minimum protein intake of 60 grams daily, with a common range of up to 1.5 grams per kilogram of ideal body weight per day. In certain high-need individuals, the requirement can climb as high as 2.1 grams/kg if advised by care professionals.
- Sufficient protein helps maintain lean body mass during rapid weight loss and speeds post-surgical healing.
- Achieving these protein targets with natural foods alone is challenging. Early on, most patients rely on liquid protein supplements (roughly 30 grams/day) to bridge intake gaps and maintain strength.

In the context of each recovery stage, gelatin offers unique advantages: it supports hydration, can be fortified with protein, and is gentle on the digestive tract, matching the body's reduced digestive and absorptive capacity following surgery.

The Role of Gelatin: Medically Favored for Hydration and Protein Delivery

Gelatin stands out as a preferred snack and hydration aid after bariatric surgery for several reasons. Its smooth texture and low residue make it easy to tolerate when the stomach is most sensitive. As a clear liquid when dissolved and set, unflavored or sugar-free gelatin products are suitable in the earliest dietary stage. As recovery progresses, gelatin becomes a versatile vehicle for delivering supplemental protein when fortified with specialized protein powders or clear protein supplements.

Medically, gelatin offers:

- High digestibility, which minimizes mechanical strain on the surgical site and lowers the chance of severe food intolerance or vomiting.
- Readily adjustable portion sizes to accommodate the significantly reduced gastric capacity of post-surgical patients.
- The opportunity for easy fortification: by dissolving flavorless powdered proteins in the liquid before setting, each serving of gelatin can contribute meaningfully to daily protein targets without causing taste fatigue.
- Hydration support: Substantial water is used in most gelatin recipes, and each serving counts toward daily

fluid intake, a significant challenge for many recovering patients.

Gelatin snacks can also reduce feelings of deprivation, offering a familiar texture and subtle sweetness without the risks posed by sugary foods, a critical point for avoiding dumping syndrome, which is precipitated by rapid stomach emptying of high-sugar or high-fat foods.

Sugar-Free and Protein-Enriched Gelatin Taxonomy for Bariatric Diets

To maximize the benefits of gelatin while avoiding common post-surgical pitfalls, opt for specific formulations:

Sugar-Free Gelatin

- Commercially available sugar-free gelatins (varieties such as lemon, lime, or mixed berry) contain non-caloric sweeteners and are free from table sugar. These are safe for all phases from clear liquids onward.
- When selecting commercial products, confirm the absence of sugar alcohols or artificial sweeteners that might provoke intolerance for sensitive stomachs.
- For homemade gelatin, use unflavored gelatin sheets or powder, adding permitted flavor extracts, natural fruit infusions, or low-calorie flavor drops for variety.

Protein-Enriched Gelatin

- Some ready-to-eat medical nutrition products are formulated specifically for bariatric patients, delivering significant protein per serving in a pre-gelled, sugar-free format.
- DIY protein gelatin snacks can be made by dissolving measured doses of approved clear liquid protein supplements (or flavorless protein powders) into the hot liquid as you prepare the gelatin. The resulting snack is both hydrating and protein-rich, with textures and flavors tailored to individual preference and stage.
- Patients may also blend in additional nutrients, such as pureed fruits, puddings, or Greek yogurt, as they advance to later recovery stages (only after clearance from the medical team).

Bariatric Diet Stage Progression Table: When and How to Introduce Gelatin

The decision of when and how to introduce each type of gelatin product follows strict stage criteria set by your bariatric team. Below is a summary guide mapping out safe incorporation of gelatin-based snacks throughout the diet progression:

Table 1: Bariatric Diet Stage Progression Table

Diet Stage	Permit Sugar-Free Gelatin?	Permit Protein-Enriched Gelatin?	Typical Add-ins
Clear Liquid	Yes, if sugar-free	Yes, if clear and sugar-free	None
Full Liquid	Yes	Yes, can increase protein/fiber	Flavorings; little to no solids
Pureed	Yes	Yes	Pureed soft fruits, non-fat dairy, as tolerated
Soft	Yes	Yes	Soft fruits, yogurt, soft grains (advanced)
Regular	Yes	Yes	All as tolerated, including higher protein mix-ins

Clinical criteria for safely introducing gelatin at each stage include:

- No vomiting, nausea, or intolerance of current textures and fluid volumes for at least 24-48 hours.
- Meeting minimum daily fluid and protein goals.
- Stepwise, incremental serving sizes and careful observation for digestive symptoms after any new gelatin product is added to the meal plan.

Monitor for signs of intolerance (bloating, cramps, excessive sweetness sensitivity) and revert to the previous stage if issues arise. Always coordinate with your bariatric dietitian to tailor the introduction to your individual needs and tolerance thresholds.

Weekly Meal Plan: Gelatin-Based Snacks and Desserts

To illustrate how gelatin snacks can be smoothly integrated into daily routines, consider the following sample weekly snack plan for various recovery stages (portion and stage-appropriate):

- ***Day 1 (Clear Liquid)***: Sugar-free lemon gelatin, 2 oz serving, mid-morning and afternoon
- ***Day 2 (Clear Liquid)***: Sugar-free unflavored gelatin with a splash of orange essence, 2 oz serving, midday
- ***Day 3 (Full Liquid)***: Protein-enriched berry gelatin, 2 oz snack after evening meal
- ***Day 4 (Full Liquid)***: Commercial protein gelatin, 2 oz snack; sugar-free lime gelatin, afternoon
- ***Day 5 (Pureed)***: Homemade protein gelatin blended with pureed peaches, 3 oz dessert
- ***Day 6 (Soft)***: Protein-rich gelatin parfait with a small spoon of low-fat Greek yogurt, 3 oz, evening
- ***Day 7 (Regular)***: Protein-enriched mixed berry gelatin cubes, 3 oz with optional unsweetened fruit toppings, lunchbox snack

Always adjust exact serving sizes and frequency to your surgeon's or dietitian's stage-specific recommendations.

Space snacks at least 1-2 hours apart from main meals to ensure adequate nutrient absorption and to avoid discomfort from overfilling the pouch.

Understanding the staged bariatric diet progression, meeting hydration and protein targets, and leveraging the unique advantages of gelatin snacks are the foundations of early and long-term recovery after bariatric surgery. Sugar-free, protein-enriched gelatin occupies a valuable niche as a safe, enjoyable, and easy-to-tolerate treat from the very first clear liquid days through to maintenance.

By choosing appropriate commercial or homemade options and respecting clinical progression criteria, you can optimize healing, preserve lean mass, and support a smoother transition to a balanced, sustainable post-bariatric way of eating.

In the following chapters, you'll find practical shopping, preparation, and recipe guidance, ensuring gelatin treats remain a safe, satisfying staple throughout your bariatric journey. Remember, always check with your bariatric care team before introducing any new gelatin product into your post-surgical diet.

Gelatin Product Selection for Bariatric Patients

Choosing gelatin products after bariatric surgery involves more than taste or convenience; it requires careful attention to product safety, nutrient value, and stage-specific recovery needs. This chapter outlines how to select suitable gelatin products for each phase of bariatric recovery, whether you use ready-made products, make your own, or enhance them with protein supplements.

You'll find medically grounded checklists, precise evaluation criteria, and prompts to help you shop and prepare gelatin responsibly and under your bariatric team's guidance.

Requirements Checklist for Safe Gelatin Products

Every gelatin dessert or snack in a post-bariatric meal plan must meet strict criteria. After surgery, the stomach (and sometimes the small intestine) is especially sensitive, so selected products should not trigger dumping syndrome, should support healing, and should contribute to essential protein intake without introducing new risks.

When reviewing commercial or DIY gelatin, use this checklist:

1. ***Sugar-Free***: Only choose gelatin with no added sugars, as sugar can trigger dumping syndrome (rapid stomach emptying, nausea, cramping, diarrhea). Check for "sugar-free" labels and absence of table sugar, corn syrup, honey, or juice concentrates.
2. ***Low-Calorie***: Pick products with no more than 10-20 calories per serving (without protein additions) to avoid excess calorie intake during early recovery.
3. ***High-Protein***: From the full liquid stage onward, favor gelatin snacks fortified with protein or those that mix easily with approved protein supplements. Achieving daily protein targets (often at least 60g) is crucial for muscle maintenance and healing, especially after bariatric surgery.
4. ***Allergen Awareness***: Gelatin is usually animal-based, but some versions may have egg, milk, or nuts. Always read labels for allergens, especially with food sensitivities or history of post-op intolerance.
5. ***Artificial Sweetener Tolerability***: Most sugar-free gelatins contain artificial sweeteners (aspartame, sucralose, acesulfame K). While generally tolerated, these can cause GI symptoms in some. Start with small

amounts and consult your dietitian to confirm which sweeteners are best for you.

6. ***Texture and Consistency***: Gelatin should match your current dietary stage and be free of large fruit chunks or nuts until you're on a soft or regular diet.

Comparison Table: Ready-to-Eat, Mix-at-Home, Unflavored Gelatin Proteins

Gelatin options for bariatric patients typically fall into three main categories, each with strengths and limitations for safety, protein content, and convenience:

Table 2: Comparison Table

Product Type	Sugar-Free	Protein-Enriched Option	Additive Control	Supplement Compatibility	Best Stage Use	Key Considerations
Ready-to-Eat Retail	Often	Sometimes (medical)	Low	Limited	Clear/ Full Liquid, Maintenance	Convenient, but usually low-protein; some have hidden sugars/thickeners
Mix-at-Home (Flavored)	Usually	Yes (add powder/liquid)	Moderate	High	Full Liquid onward	Easy to enrich with protein; check for sweeteners and colorings
Unflavored Gelatin	Always	Yes (add powder/liquid)	High	High	All Stages	Most customizable; suitable for early phases and tailored to needs

Ready-to-eat retail gelatins (like store-bought sugar-free cups) are convenient but generally low in protein unless marked for medical use. Some specialty brands sell pre-made, bariatric-targeted protein gelatins, though availability may be limited.

Mix-at-home flavored gelatin powders are often available sugar-free and can be enriched with protein from the full liquid stage onward. Always verify flavors and colorings for tolerability and avoid contraindicated ingredients.

Pure unflavored gelatin (powder or sheets) gives you maximal control on sweeteners, colors, or flavors by default. Combine it with clear broths, sugar-free drink mixes, or protein supplements to match your dietary stage and needs, improving both safety and flexibility.

Criteria for Reading and Evaluating Ingredient Labels

Reading ingredient labels is essential after bariatric surgery, as even "sugar-free" products may contain ingredients that cause issues.

Steps for label evaluation:

1. ***Ingredients List***: Confirm absence of sugar, corn syrup, glucose syrup, honey, fruit juice concentrate, or maltodextrin these are not safe in early stages.
2. ***Sweeteners***: Use only approved non-nutritive sweeteners (e.g., stevia, sucralose, aspartame); avoid excess sugar alcohols (sorbitol, xylitol) unless you know they agree with you.

3. ***Coloring Agents***: Avoid artificial colors if you're sensitive, especially early after surgery. Choose colorless/unflavored gelatin if needed.
4. ***Protein Fortification***: If "protein-added," check the protein source (whey, collagen, egg white) to confirm it's compatible with your diet.
5. ***Allergen and Safety Statements***: Look for warnings about milk, eggs, soy, or nuts. Skip any product missing a full list of ingredients, as sensitivity is common.
6. ***Serving Size/Preparation Directions***: Ensure serving size fits your dietitian's guidelines, often just 2-3 ounces in early recovery.

If a label is unclear, contact the manufacturer or ask your provider to review the product.

Framework for Choosing Protein Powders or Supplements for Gelatin

To boost daily protein intake, pairing gelatin with bariatric-suitable protein supplements is highly effective. Use this checklist when selecting a protein for homemade or customized gelatin snacks:

- ***Protein Source***: Choose clear, tasteless, high-quality isolates such as whey isolate, hydrolyzed collagen, or medically formulated clear protein drinks approved for bariatric use. Avoid those with added sugar, fat, or irritants.

- ***Mixability***: Confirm the protein powder dissolves well in cool or slightly warm liquids to avoid gritty or clumpy textures.
- ***Concentration***: Look for at least 10-20g protein per serving to help meet daily targets efficiently.
- ***Additive Profile***: Select powders with minimal additives; reject those with excess flavorings, colorings, or bulking fibers not cleared by your care team.
- ***Allergen Status***: Ensure the powder is free from any triggers (e.g., lactose, gluten, soy) per your dietary restrictions.
- ***Supplement Compatibility***: If you take vitamins/minerals, ensure your protein powder won't negatively interact with other supplements in your gelatin recipe.

Always test a new protein with a small gelatin batch to check texture and tolerability. If texture is off or you react poorly, seek other brands or ask your dietitian for suggestions.

Key Questions for Confirming Surgeon or Dietitian Approval

Approval from your bariatric care team is vital before trying any new gelatin product or formulation. Discuss these questions with your provider:

1. Is this product appropriate for my current diet stage?
2. Does it fit my specific protein, calorie, and carbohydrate limits?
3. Are its sweeteners and flavorings safe for my health history and past tolerances?
4. Should I use caution with its protein source due to any allergies?
5. Is it compatible with my supplements, meal replacements, or medications?
6. What is the safe portion size per snack/serving right now?
7. What symptoms (gas, bloating, upset stomach) should I watch for as warning signs?
8. How should I track my body's response to any new gelatin products?

Bariatric teams always recommend a gradual approach and close monitoring for signs of intolerance or dumping syndrome. If unsure, bring the packaging or product to your next appointment for review.

Choosing the right gelatin products can enhance your recovery by offering hydration, flavor, and crucial protein as you progress through dietary stages. By following safety checklists, understanding ingredient labels and supplement interactions, and involving your care team with every new product, you'll set yourself up for smoother, safer recovery.

Armed with these strategies, you'll confidently navigate sugar-free and protein-enhanced gelatin selections. Always prioritize tolerability, customization, and ongoing medical oversight, ensuring every gelatin snack serves your recovery and well-being.

Safe Preparation Techniques for Post-Surgical Needs

Preparing gelatin snacks and desserts after bariatric surgery involves more than following a typical recipe. Every aspect of temperature, mixing technique, handling, and storage matters for your safety, healing, and nutritional success.

This chapter provides a complete, practical roadmap for making sugar-free, protein-first gelatins tailored to post-surgery needs. Whether you're still on clear liquids or transitioning to regular foods, these preparation strategies build a safe, medically sound foundation for enjoying gelatin at every step.

Temperature and Mixing Dos and Don'ts to Prevent Lumping and Maintain Nutrient Integrity

Crafting homemade gelatin that's both smooth and nutritionally potent is a balancing act especially when incorporating protein supplements or avoiding common mishaps like lumps. Here are essential temperature and mixing guidelines for the best results and maximum nutrient preservation.

1. ***Dissolve Gelatin Properly***: Always start by sprinkling unflavored gelatin powder over a small amount of cold liquid (water or approved clear broth). Let it sit for a couple of minutes until it blooms; this ensures even hydration and prevents unwanted lumps.
2. ***Use Correct Water Temperatures***: After blooming, add very hot but not boiling water (typically 120–140°F or about 50–60°C) to dissolve the gelatin fully. Boiling water can scorch added protein or sweeteners, degrading nutrients and affecting taste.
3. ***Gentle Mixing***: If adding protein powder, dissolve it separately in cool or room-temperature water first. Once well mixed with no visible clumps, fold it gently into the dissolved gelatin base. Vigorous or prolonged stirring with hot liquids can denature protein, harm texture, or create air bubbles. For best results, use a small whisk or immersion blender on low speed, avoiding over-mixing.
4. ***Add Sweeteners and Flavors at the Right Time***: Add artificial sweeteners, extracts, or zero-calorie syrups only after the gelatin has dissolved and the mixture has cooled slightly (but is still liquid), preserving their potency and preventing separation.
5. ***Avoid Rapid Temperature Changes***: Never put hot gelatin mixture directly into the refrigerator; instead,

allow it to cool on the counter until lukewarm. Sudden chilling can cause separation or a rubbery layer. Once cooled, pour into containers and refrigerate.

6. ***Maintain Protein Integrity***: If using a whey isolate or hydrolyzed collagen, keep the mixing temperature moderate never exceed 140°F (60°C) to protect protein structure and maximize absorption. This supports lean body mass preservation, which is especially crucial in the post-bariatric phase, where meeting protein targets is challenging.

Portion Size, Serving Texture, and Food Safety Handling Rules

After surgery, your stomach's reduced capacity and sensitivity to texture mean careful control over portion size, consistency, and hygiene is crucial.

Portion Size Guidelines

- ***Clear/Full Liquid Phase***: Serve gelatin in small 2 oz (60 mL) portions, matching your care team's guidance and allowing for slow, mindful consumption.
- ***Pureed/Soft Foods Phase***: Increase portions slightly to 3–4 oz (90–120 mL) per snack, only as tolerated.
- ***Regular Foods Phase***: 4 oz (120 mL) per serving remains typical, ensuring protein or calorie intake goals are not exceeded.

These sizes help prevent overfilling your pouch, reducing the risk of nausea, regurgitation, or vomiting common issues in early recovery.

Serving Texture Expectations

- ***Early Stages***: Gelatin should be clear, entirely smooth, and free from any solid or chewy inclusions.
- ***Pureed/Post-Pureed***: Texture may be a bit thicker, but still without any chunks. Protein-fortified gelatins must dissolve easily on the tongue without grittiness.
- ***Maintenance/Regular***: At this point, some fruit puree or very soft inclusions may be added but always confirm with your care team.

Food Safety Rules

1. Always use clean, sanitized utensils to prevent bacterial contamination. Post-surgical patients, especially those with temporary immune suppression from rapid weight loss or reduced food intake, are at higher risk of foodborne illness.
2. Prepare gelatin in small, single-use batches to minimize time in the fridge and maximize freshness.
3. Refrigerate gelatins immediately after portioning. Never leave prepared snacks at room temperature for longer than 30 minutes.
4. Discard any gelatin with an off smell, unusual color, or separation.

5. Do not consume any gelatin that has been left uncovered in the fridge or beyond its safe storage period (usually 3–5 days).

Implementation of a Contamination-Avoidance Checklist

Immunocompromised patients common immediately post-bariatric surgery due to altered nutritional and metabolic states must be extra vigilant about contamination risk. Here's a streamlined checklist to prevent issues:

- ***Wash Hands Thoroughly***: Before prepping or portioning, wash hands for at least 20 seconds.
- ***Sanitize Surfaces***: Clean countertops, cutting boards, utensils, and mixing bowls with hot, soapy water before and after use.
- ***Use Food-Safe Gloves***: When portioning large batches or if you have any healing wounds on your hands.
- ***Select Single-Serve Containers***: Prevents contamination from multiple openings or serving.
- ***Store Separately***: Keep protein-enriched and non-enriched batches separate in the fridge to reduce cross-contact.
- ***Refrigerate Immediately***: Place all prepared gelatin in the fridge within 15–30 minutes of pouring.

- ***Label and Date***: Mark containers with the preparation date and intended recipient if several people share a refrigerator.
- ***Discard on Schedule***: Never eat gelatin past the safe storage period even if it appears visually fine.

If you have recently been ill, are on immunosuppressive medication, or have a history of infections, discuss additional handling precautions with your dietitian or bariatric care team.

Utensil and Container Selection for Optimal Portion Control and Recovery Ease

Selecting the right containers and utensils enhances portion control, critical in preventing overconsumption and ensuring compliance with your stage-specific dietary plan.

Best Practices for Containers

- Use small, transparent containers (2–4 oz) for clear visual tracking of portions. This prevents accidental overeating and supports your dietary goals.
- Choose containers with tight-fitting lids to prevent cross-contamination and drying out.
- Silicone molds can be helpful for unmolding single-serve portions easily, especially if wrist mobility is limited after surgery.

- For protein-enriched recipes, ensure the vessel can be sealed tightly, as these may be more prone to spoilage.

Recommended Utensils

- ***Soft silicone spatulas***: Gentle on containers and ensure protein powder is mixed in thoroughly with minimal product loss on utensils.
- ***Mini whisks or immersion blenders (low speed)***: Excellent for dispersing protein powder without creating foam or interfering with set.
- ***Medicine cups or shot glasses***: Serve as portion guides for early-stage servings.
- ***Labeling markers***: For marking container dates and contents.

Convenience tip: Pre-portion your gelatin as soon as it's poured into containers. Avoid "breaking off" servings from a larger pan, as this can make accurate tracking harder and increase contamination risk.

Visual Gelatin Preparation Step-by-Step Guide for Traditional & Protein-Enhanced Recipes

Here's a clear, stepwise process for preparing both basic and protein-fortified gelatin snacks, optimized for bariatric recovery phases:

Traditional (Basic/Sugar-Free) Gelatin Preparation

1. ***Bloom the gelatin***: Sprinkle the required amount of unflavored gelatin powder onto a small amount of cold, sugar-free fluid (such as water or allowed clear beverage), letting it stand for 2–5 minutes.
2. ***Dissolve***: Add hot (not boiling) water to the bloomed gelatin. Stir gently until completely dissolved with no visible granules.
3. ***Flavor (optional)***: Blend in zero-calorie flavor extract or allowed artificial sweetener, ensuring full dissolution.
4. ***Portion***: Pour the liquid into single-serve containers (2–4 oz for early stages).
5. ***Cool***: Let sit at room temperature until no longer hot, then refrigerate immediately.
6. ***Set***: Chill for several hours until firm. If using the full liquid stage, the goal is a gel that quivers and dissolves easily on the tongue but can be eaten with a spoon.

Protein-Enhanced Gelatin Preparation

1. Bloom gelatin as above in a small bowl.
2. Prepare protein slurry: In a separate cup, dissolve the required scoop of bariatric-approved protein powder in a small volume of room-temperature water. Stir until smooth—no lumps should remain.
3. Combine: Add the bloomed gelatin to hot (120–140°F) water and stir until dissolved. Mix in the cooled

protein slurry gently, using a small whisk or immersion blender on low to prevent foaming.

4. Add sweetener/flavors after the solution has cooled moderately (about body temperature).
5. Portion into single-serve, tightly lidded containers.
6. Refrigerate until fully set (at least 2–4 hours).

Practical Tips and Troubleshooting

- If you notice protein "clumping" or a gritty bottom layer, next time use slightly less hot water and whisk protein powder longer before adding.
- Should the gelatin set too firmly (difficult to cut with a spoon), reduce the gelatin or protein slightly for softer results, ideal for early post-op stages.
- Never attempt to freeze gelatin snacks for later use until you have reached the maintenance phase, and only if your care team has approved it freezing can radically alter texture in a way that may not be safe for your current food tolerance stage.

Safety Reminders Throughout Preparation

- Prepare only what you'll use within 3–5 days. Smaller, more frequent batches limit waste and contamination risk.
- Always use boiling water to clean and sterilize utensils and molds before use.

- When in doubt about a particular batch, err on the side of caution and discard if it appears or smells off.

Mastering safe preparation techniques for bariatric gelatin recipes is integral to your post-surgery dietary success. By carefully controlling temperatures, portion sizes, and handling, as well as using the right tools and preparation steps, you're providing your body with safe, satisfying, and stage-appropriate nutrition. Protein-enhanced gelatins, in particular, deliver the essential building blocks your body needs to heal and maintain muscle, with the gentle texture and flavor variety that support compliance and enjoyment at every step.

Keep these techniques and safety guidelines close at hand each week as you batch prepare gelatin snacks and desserts. These routines, coupled with regular review by your bariatric dietitian, help ensure each gelatin treat is as safe and beneficial as it is delicious and comforting.

Stage 1 and 2 Recipes: Clear and Full Liquid Gelatin Snacks

Recovery after bariatric surgery begins with the clear and full liquid stages, where the texture and composition of what you eat are strictly controlled for your safety and optimal healing. Gelatin-based snacks offer a unique solution during these phases, providing hydration, customizable flavor, and an approachable way to begin regaining your protein intake.

This chapter gives you a clear, medically responsible framework for preparing gelatin snacks aligned with clinical guidelines, and equips you with practical recipes, adjustment methods, and troubleshooting pointers to support your journey from clear liquids to fuller, more nourishing choices.

Gelatin Recipe Framework for Clear and Full Liquid Stages

The first stages after surgery clear liquid and full liquid require foods and fluids to be easy on your healing stomach, free of solids, and simple to digest. During these phases, gelatin serves several vital roles:

- ***Hydration support***: Gelatin snacks are predominantly water, making them ideal for supporting your daily fluid targets, which is crucial early on when swallowing or tolerating large volumes is difficult.
- ***Texture safety***: Properly prepared gelatin is smooth, dissolves easily in the mouth, and can be made soft enough for even the most sensitive healing pouch. This quality is especially important when regurgitation, nausea, or vomiting are risks if you advance food textures too quickly.
- ***Nutrition delivery***: With careful recipe modification, gelatin can serve as a vehicle for protein from liquid supplements, helping you close the gap toward early macronutrient targets that would otherwise be challenging with natural foods alone.

The key to safe and effective gelatin snacks in these early stages is formula flexibility: adjusting the ratio of water to gelatin to protein supplement to create "hydro-gel" snacks that deliver hydration, gentle satiety, and critical nutrients in a tiny, easily managed portion.

The foundation of every recipe at this stage includes:

1. ***Unflavored gelatin powder*** (for maximum ingredient control).
2. ***Water or permitted clear liquid*** (broth, diluted sugar-free juice).
3. ***Sugar-free flavoring*** (see next section for guidance).

4. ***Bariatric-formulated liquid protein supplement*** (isolate or hydrolyzed for best tolerance and mixing).

As you progress from clear liquids (stage 1) to full liquids (stage 2), the consistency and protein content can be cautiously increased, always following your clinic's timeline and tolerances.

Sugar-Free Flavoring Agents and Liquid Protein Add-In Guidelines for Stage 1/2 Safety

In the first postoperative weeks, strict sugar avoidance is a medical priority. Simple sugars and high-calorie additives can cause dangerous dumping syndrome or reactive hypoglycemia due to the rapid delivery of nutrients to your intestine. Flavor and sweetness are still important, but they should come from sources that do not contribute sugar calories or risk gut discomfort.

Safe flavoring options include:

- ***Liquid stevia or sucralose-based drops***: Read ingredient lists carefully for hidden sugars.
- ***Powdered or liquid "water enhancer" drops***: Opt for zero-calorie, sugar-free products only.
- ***Natural or artificial extracts (vanilla, lemon, orange, almond)***: Use sparingly, confirm with your care team.

- ***Sugar-free syrups (if allowed by your dietitian)***: Only include syrups certified safe for bariatric patients and those free of maltitol or high-risk sweeteners prone to causing bloating or diarrhea.

For color and variety, tiny drops of natural food coloring can be used once cleared by your dietitian.

Liquid protein add-in guidelines:

- Only use protein supplements recommended or approved by your bariatric team.
- Opt for whey protein isolate, hydrolyzed collagen, or medical-grade clear liquid protein designed for postoperative use.
- Avoid products with added sugars, fillers, or problematic artificial sweeteners.
- Mix and dissolve protein separately before combining with gelatin (as described in Chapter 3) to prevent clumping and ensure even distribution.
- Carefully track the amount per batch so you know exactly how much protein is in each serving.

The target for total daily protein intake is typically at least 60 grams per day, with small, frequent servings throughout the day preferred over large doses, especially in the first several weeks. Protein-enriched gelatin can help you meet incremental targets in just a few spoonfuls per snack, while also boosting satiety and supporting recovery.

Hydration/Protein Ratio Adjustment Table for Balancing Fluid Intake and Minimum Macronutrient Needs

As you construct your meals and snacks from gelatin, it's crucial to maintain the correct balance between hydration (fluid) and protein content so you do not inadvertently under- or overshoot these goals. Too little fluid can worsen dehydration, while too much protein in a single snack may cause intolerance or poor dissolution.

Below is a practical adjustment guide for one batch (yielding four 2-oz servings, or about 240 mL total):

Table 3: Hydration/Protein Ratio Adjustment Table

Stage	Water or Clear Fluid	Protein Supple-ment* (per batch)	Unflavored Gelatin	Flavoring	Note
Clear	220 mL (scant cup)	5–10 g (medical-grade liquid)	1 packet (7 g)	Sugar-free drop	Start at lower end; avoid excess
Full	200 mL	10–15 g	1½ packets (10 g)	As above	Gradually increase as tolerated

Use only protein products approved for bariatric use; measure carefully.

- For hydration, keeping each gelatin serving "soft" and easy to dissolve the fluid amount should allow the snack to nearly melt on the tongue, especially in the clear liquid stage.

- For protein: begin conservatively. If you experience any chalky texture, heaviness, or intolerance, slightly decrease the protein in your next batch or switch to a more soluble supplement.

General tip: Never attempt to fulfill your entire daily protein quota via gelatin alone, but use it as one component in a rotation with clear protein drinks, broth, and other permitted liquids.

Three Clinically Compliant Recipes for Clear, Protein-Infused Gelatins with Preparation Details

Below are three recipe templates tailored for safety and compliance during stages 1 and 2. Each makes four 2-oz servings to adjust batch size if preparing for a single day or desired number of snack servings.

Basic Clear Protein Gelatin

Ingredients:

- 220 mL cold water, divided
- 1 packet (7 g) unflavored gelatin powder
- 2–3 drops sugar-free flavor extract (such as lemon, orange, or raspberry)
- 10 g bariatric-approved clear liquid protein supplement

Instructions:

1. In a small bowl, sprinkle gelatin powder over 60 mL cold water. Let sit (bloom) 3–5 min.
2. Meanwhile, dissolve protein supplement in a separate 40 mL water, stirring until absolutely smooth.
3. Heat the remaining 120 mL water to steaming (but not boiling, max 140°F or 60°C).
4. Pour hot water over bloomed gelatin; stir gently to dissolve.
5. Once gelatin is dissolved and mixture is below 110°F (about body temp), add protein slurry and flavor drops.
6. Divide among four clean, lidded 2-oz containers. Cool until set (at least 2–3 hours).

Citrus-Infused Hydration Gel

Ingredients:

- 200 mL clear, sugar-free lemon/lime electrolyte beverage
- 1½ packets (10 g) unflavored gelatin
- ½ tsp sugar-free lemon extract (if desired)
- 12 g clear whey isolate protein (ensure it dissolves well)

Instructions:

1. Prepare gelatin with 50 mL cold electrolyte drink, let bloom 5 min.
2. Dissolve protein isolate in another 50 mL cold electrolyte beverage, stirring to remove lumps.
3. Heat remaining 100 mL until steaming; combine with bloomed gelatin.
4. Once mixture is warm but not hot, add protein and extract.
5. Portion into clean containers; refrigerate until fully set and jiggly.

Berry Protein Gel Cubes

Ingredients:

- 210 mL cold water
- 1 packet (7 g) unflavored gelatin
- ¼ tsp sugar-free berry flavoring
- 1–2 drops liquid food coloring (optional, confirmed safe)
- 8 g clear liquid hydrolyzed collagen protein

Instructions:

1. Bloom gelatin in 50 mL cold water; let stand 3 min.
2. Dissolve collagen in a separate 40 mL water; stir vigorously.
3. Heat remainder of water to just below boiling, add to bloomed gelatin and mix.
4. When mixture cools to touch, add protein solution, flavor, and coloring.
5. Pour into silicone ice cube tray for easy demolding; chill until gelatin is delicate but holds together.

All recipes should yield a soft, clear, and completely smooth gel never rubbery or gritty. Discard any batches that set unevenly or have protein “sediment” visible at the bottom.

Troubleshooting Texture Problems, Such as Excessive Firmness or Improper Setting

The most common issues with homemade protein-enhanced gelatin snacks are over-firm gels, runny or unset textures, and gritty or layered results. Here’s how to address and prevent these challenges:

1. **Too Firm (Rubbery, Hard to Spoon):**
    - Decrease the amount of gelatin powder by ¼ packet at a time.
    - If using higher-protein content, dilute the batch slightly or use a more soluble protein supplement.
    - Avoid chilling too quickly; rapid temperature drops can toughen the gel.

2. **Not Setting (Stays Liquid or Syrupy):**
    - Check that water temperature is hot enough to dissolve the gelatin fully (but not boiling).
    - Ensure gelatin is fresh, not expired and has not absorbed moisture from storage.
    - Use the recommended gelatin-to-water ratio; under-measuring gelatin is a frequent cause.

3. **Protein Layering or Grit:**
    - Always dissolve protein powder completely in cold or room-temperature liquid before combining with gelatin.
    - Add the protein solution only when gelatin mix has cooled slightly after dissolving, not when piping hot.
    - Avoid over-stirring or aggressive whisking, which can create bubbles and separate layers.
    - Try a finer, more soluble medical-grade protein if persistent issues occur.
4. **Separation After Setting:**
    - Provides a signal that temperature transfer was too rapid, or that protein and gelatin weren't fully homogenized before chilling.
    - Next time, allow the gelatin-protein mixture to cool to room temperature before refrigeration.
5. **Cloudiness:**

    Mild haze is normal with some protein supplements, but milky appearance may indicate improper mixing. Dissolve all ingredients fully before chilling.

Always remember, early post-bariatric phases require utmost caution: if you cannot achieve a smooth, soft, easily dissolving gelatin texture, scale back the protein or consult with your dietitian for permissible commercial options until you master the mixing process.

Weekly Meal Plan: Stage 1 and 2 Gelatin Snacks

Here's a sample snack plan integrating your newly mastered gelatin recipes into a compliant liquid-phase intake. Each day features 2–3 gelatin servings among your overall liquid plan:

Day 1

- Breakfast: 2 oz citrus-infused hydration gel
- Mid-morning: 2 oz basic protein gelatin
- Afternoon: 4 oz clear broth

Day 2

- Breakfast: 2 oz berry protein gel cube
- Late morning: 2 oz clear protein drink
- Evening: 2 oz basic protein gelatin

Day 3

Spread your servings throughout the day, rotating flavors. For example: 2 oz citrus gel in the afternoon, 2 oz basic protein at dinner.

Continue alternating recipes to avoid flavor fatigue and support your daily hydration and protein goals. Remember: total daily liquid volume from all sources (gelatin, broth, drinks) should match your care team's recommendations to avoid dehydration.

Using this structured approach to gelatin snacks in the first two post-surgery stages provides both medical safety and comfort. With careful planning and adjustment, you can achieve satisfying hydration, meet minimum protein requirements, and build confidence in food prep all while being gentle on your healing digestive system. Your attention to detail now sets the stage for more varied and substantial foods as you progress through each phase of your bariatric recovery.

Stage 3 Pureed to Stage 4 Soft: Transitional Gelatin-Based Blends

Transitioning from a liquid-based post-bariatric diet to pureed and soft foods is a critical step in your recovery journey. It is a time of reintroducing variety, testing food tolerance, and gradually building the confidence and skills necessary for lifelong dietary changes.

During these phases Stage 3 (Pureed) and Stage 4 (Soft) gelatin remains a uniquely valuable ingredient. It not only provides a familiar texture base as you shift away from clear liquids but also serves as a gentle carrier for new flavors, nutrients, and protein sources appropriate to your expanding dietary palette.

Criteria for Integrating Pureed Fruits or Dairy with Gelatin for Stage 3

As you move into Stage 3, your healthcare team will guide you in cautiously incorporating slightly thicker textures and more nutrient-dense foods. At this point, integrating pureed fruits or select dairy products with your gelatin provides a safe, customizable way to introduce flavor, minimal fiber, and a creamy consistency, all while keeping your snack gentle and easy to digest. However, careful attention to food choice, sugar content, and texture is essential.

To safely integrate pureed fruits or dairy with gelatin at Stage 3:

- Only use fruits and dairy cleared by your surgeon or bariatric dietitian. Typically, low-acid, seedless, and soft fruits (such as banana, canned peaches in juice, or cooked apples) are preferred, and only in pureed, lump-free form.
- Select plain, non-fat Greek yogurt, lactose-free quark, or soft ricotta for dairy options. Avoid full-fat, full-sugar yogurts and any dairy with pieces, rinds, or inclusions.
- Ensure all fruit purees are unsweetened with no added sugars or syrups.
- Limit total puree/dairy blend amount to no more than half the total weight of your gelatin recipe to maintain a soft, safe gel consistency.
- Always use sugar-free gelatin bases, preferably unflavored, to prevent excess sweetness and reduce the risk of dumping syndrome or reactive hypoglycemia, both of which are risks in the post-bariatric context when simple sugars are introduced too early.

- For protein, continue to incorporate your approved liquid or powder supplement, dissolving fully before adding to the mix. Protein requirement remains at least 60 grams per day even at this stage, best accomplished through frequent, small meals and snacks.
- Test any new addition (fruit, dairy, or protein powder variant) in a tiny initial serving, monitoring closely for satiety cues, intolerance, or discomfort before proceeding with regular use.

Safe List of Blend-In Foods by Stage with Contraindicated Items Clearly Marked

To help you confidently and safely expand your gelatin-based creations, here's a stage-specific list of blend-in options, with contraindicated items highlighted for clarity. Always check for updates from your care team before making changes.

Stage 3 (Pureed Foods) – Permitted Blend-ins:

- Pureed banana (small amount, fully smooth, no lumps)
- Pureed canned peaches (in juice, drained, no sugar added)
- Cooked, peeled pureed apple or pear (unsweetened)
- Plain, non-fat Greek yogurt (fully smooth, no fruit bits or added sugar)
- Lactose-free low-fat ricotta or cottage cheese (whipped to smooth)
- Silken tofu (blended until creamy)

- Bariatric-approved liquid or hydrolyzed protein supplement

Contraindicated at Stage 3:

- Raw or high-fiber fruits (berries with seeds, pineapple, mango)
- Dried fruits or fruit products with added sugar
- Full-fat, sweetened, or whole-milk yogurts
- Cheeses or dairy with pieces, crusts, or herbs
- Nuts, seeds, or any "crunchy" garnishes
- Unapproved protein bars or powders (those not specifically recommended for bariatric use)

Stage 4 (Soft Foods) – Permitted Blend-ins (in addition to above):

- Mashed avocado (limit portion due to fat content)
- Seedless, cooked soft fruit (ripe peeled pears)
- Small amounts of soft, smooth nut butter (only if cleared by your team)
- Whipped light cream cheese (ensure tolerability, limit fat)
- Soft-cooked, pureed pumpkin or squash (unsweetened)
- Smooth, small-curd cottage cheese (if extremely well tolerated)
- Gradually introduce slightly textured fruits if advised, always starting with a very small portion and monitoring response

Contraindicated at Stage 4:

- Tough fruit skins or seeds
- Hard/raw vegetables, chunky salsa
- All granola or toasted toppings
- Chocolate chips, candy, or confections
- Whole nuts or seeds

Remember, even as you progress, vigilance for adverse reactions and portion size control are key.

Stepwise Recipe Template for Single-Serve, Soft-Texture Gelatin Parfaits or Mousse

Creating a soft-texture gelatin parfait or mousse is an efficient, manageable way to meet taste and nutrition needs during your transition to soft foods. Here is a foundational template that you can personalize within your permitted blend-in list.

Single-Serve Protein Gelatin Parfait (Stage 3/4)

Ingredients:

- 1 teaspoon (2.5 g) unflavored gelatin powder
- 2 tablespoons (30 mL) cold water
- ¼ cup (60 mL) non-fat plain Greek yogurt (or approved soft dairy)
- 2–3 tablespoons (30–45 mL) pureed fruit (banana, canned peach, or allowed fruit)
- 1 scoop (as directed) unflavored or mild-flavored protein powder or 10 g clear protein liquid
- 1–2 drops sugar-free extract or sweetener (optional)

Instructions:

1. Sprinkle gelatin over cold water in a small bowl; let “bloom” 3–5 minutes.
2. While gelatin blooms, thoroughly blend fruit puree and yogurt until completely smooth and lump-free.
3. If using protein powder, dissolve in a small splash of water (per manufacturer instructions) to avoid clumping.
4. Gently heat the bloomed gelatin mixture microwave in short bursts or set the bowl in hot water just until it dissolves (do not boil).

5. Quickly combine dissolved gelatin with the yogurt-fruit-protein blend, mixing until fully smooth. Add flavor extract or sweetener as needed.
6. Pour mixture into a single-serve glass or ramekin. Tap gently to level. Refrigerate at least 2 hours until softly set.
7. Serve chilled. The final texture should be soft-set, spoonable, and completely smooth (never rubbery or grainy).

To create a mousse effect for Stage 4, simply fold 1 tablespoon of whipped, light cream cheese or plain, low-fat ricotta into the yogurt-fruit base before chilling.

This base makes a gentle, protein-first snack or dessert that supports both your nutritional goals and safe advancement through the refeeding stages.

Flavor-Pairing Chart for Gentle Transitions Between Meal Stages

Changing meal texture doesn't have to mean losing flavor variety. The following chart provides safe, appealing combinations that introduce new tastes while maintaining careful stage progression. Each pairing is aligned with tolerated ingredients and advances variety as your diet broadens.

Stage 3 (Pureed)

- Plain Greek yogurt + pureed banana + vanilla extract
- Pureed canned peach + unflavored gelatin + almond extract
- Pureed cooked pear + yogurt + cinnamon
- Silken tofu + strawberry-flavored sugar-free extract (if cleared)

Stage 4 (Soft)

- Greek yogurt + mashed avocado + lime or lemon zest (very small amount)
- Soft ricotta + peach puree + ginger or cinnamon
- Low-fat cottage cheese + pureed pumpkin + nutmeg
- Whipped light cream cheese + pureed apple + sugar-free caramel syrup

Begin with conservative portions when introducing any new combination, and always monitor for signs of intolerance or discomfort.

Common Transition Difficulties and Adjustment Tactics for Advancing Safely

Advancing through Stages 3 and 4 often brings both excitement and unexpected hurdles. The body is adjusting not only to new textures but also to the altered digestion and nutrient absorption patterns following surgery. Here are the most frequent challenges and practical solutions for safely navigating this transitional period with gelatin-based blends:

1. **Intolerance to Texture or Unfamiliar Ingredients:**
    - Signs include bloating, nausea, fullness, or regurgitation after eating.
    - Solution: Downshift to a smoother or more liquid consistency for several days before attempting blended or soft versions again. Use only single-ingredient experiment batches so you can easily identify your body's responses.
2. **Dumping Syndrome or Hypoglycemic Symptoms:**
    - Can be prompted by hidden sugars, too-large portions, or rushed fluid intake.
    - Solution: Vigilantly avoid all added sugars, large fruit quantities, or syrups. Divide snacks into two to three tiny servings, separated over

several hours. Never mix your fluid intake with your snack; wait at least 30 minutes after eating before drinking, to reduce the risk.

3. **Difficulty Meeting Protein Targets:**
    - The increasing texture and taste fatigue sometimes make it harder to consistently get enough protein each day.
    - Solution: Rotate between different approved protein powders (whey, hydrolyzed collagen, or plant-based products), and experiment with approved dairy or tofu additions for variety. Always calculate and record the protein content of each batch, aiming for a minimum of 60 grams total per day, spread out through meals and snacks.

4. **Palate Fatigue:**
    - Overexposure to one flavor or texture leads to refusal.
    - Solution: Use the flavor-pairing chart to alternate tastes throughout the week. Incorporate mild spices or herbs (such as cinnamon or nutmeg) in trace amounts for a safe and gentle expansion of flavor without adding sugar or fat.

5. **Meal Progression Anxiety:**
    - It's normal to feel apprehensive about trying new textures.
    - Solution: Progress at your own pace, but in coordination with your care team. If a texture is repeatedly problematic or unpleasant, revisit a simpler blend and gradually reintroduce complexity. Stay in close communication with your dietitian about what works and what doesn't. Sometimes small ingredient adjustments make all the difference.

Weekly Meal Plan: Gelatin-Based Snacks and Desserts for Stages 3–4

Here is a sample week that flexibly integrates your gelatin-based snacks for both pureed and soft food phases. This plan rotates flavors and textures to ensure nutrient variety and compliance.

Day 1:

- AM: Greek yogurt banana parfait (Stage 3);
- PM: Unflavored gelatin with whipped cottage cheese

Day 2:

- AM: Peach-ricotta mousse (Stage 3/4);
- PM: Soft pumpkin spice gelatin (cottage cheese and pureed pumpkin)

Day 3:

- AM: Vanilla-pear gelatin blend;
- PM: Silken tofu + sugar-free strawberry extract gel

Day 4:

- AM: Creamy apple-cinnamon parfait;
- PM: Citrus-infused yogurt gel

Day 5:

- AM: Avocado-lime gelatin blend (Stage 4);
- PM: Peach-ginger mousse

Day 6:

- AM: Pumpkin-nutmeg cottage cheese gel;
- PM: Whipped ricotta and pear parfait

Day 7:

- AM: Banana-almond extract mousse;
- PM: Cinnamon-infused apple yogurt gel

Each single-serve snack delivers gentle protein, hydration, and flavor in a portion that is easily tolerated by the healing stomach. Continue to monitor your responses and adjust serving sizes and blend-ins as you advance. If any batch is not well tolerated, scale back to a previous safe stage before retrying, and always discuss new or persistent symptoms with your bariatric care team.

Transitioning safely and happily through Stages 3 and 4 is possible with careful planning, creativity, and respect for your body's signals. Using gelatin as a flexible foundation, you can explore a wide variety of satisfying and medically appropriate snacks and desserts, supporting robust recovery and setting the tone for lifelong, protein-forward eating habits.

Protein-First Gelatin Dessert Recipes for Long-Term Maintenance

As you settle into the regular dietary phase after bariatric surgery, maintaining high protein intake remains a cornerstone of your health and weight management. The initial excitement of returning to a more varied menu can sometimes be accompanied by new challenges: rekindling appetite, curbing cravings, and continually meeting your daily protein targets, all while avoiding foods that may disrupt your progress. Protein-enriched gelatin desserts represent a creative, flexible solution: a way to make high-quality protein enjoyable, convenient, and easy on your new digestive system.

High-Protein Gelatin Recipe Checklist for Routine Snack Rotation

The foundation of your protein-first dessert routine should focus on recipes that maximize your protein intake without straying into high sugar, excessive fat, or troublesome additives. Here's a detailed checklist to guide your recipe selection and ensure that each gelatin snack fits seamlessly into your maintenance eating plan:

1. Use only gelatin recipes that are sugar-free (artificial or approved non-nutritive sweeteners only) to significantly reduce the risk of dumping syndrome or reactive hypoglycemia.
2. Every serving should provide at least 10–15 grams of complete protein—this supports you in reaching the recommended 60 grams (or more, if advised by your care team) per day.
3. Select recipes that use at least one medically approved protein supplement (such as whey isolate, hydrolyzed collagen, or clear protein fluids) designed for bariatric absorption. This helps bridge the common protein gap that natural foods alone may not fill, especially in the maintenance phase.
4. Incorporate occasional rotation of both protein types and flavors to prevent palate fatigue and maintain your interest in high-protein snacks.
5. Recipes should be batch-friendly, allowing you to prepare several servings at once for easy grab-and-go snacks throughout the week. Always observe food safety rules for preparing, portioning, and storing gelatin desserts as outlined in later chapters.
6. Each new recipe or new topping should be trialed in a small, single portion at first to allow you to monitor for

tolerance and satisfaction, especially if you are trying a new protein powder, sweetener, or extract.

Regularly including these high-protein gelatin snacks in your rotation supports muscle maintenance, satisfies cravings for dessert-like foods, and keeps your recovery on course for the long term.

Approved Protein Powders and Flavor Extracts Guide for Maintenance Use

Selecting the right protein source and flavor extracts is vital for ensuring your gelatin desserts are both medically compliant and truly delicious. As you move forward into long-term maintenance, your protein supplement must be easily absorbed and low in additives or ingredients that might irritate your post-bariatric system.

Approved protein supplements often include:

- ***Whey protein isolate***: Highly absorbable, neutral taste, and ideal for mixing with both basic and flavored gelatin bases. Look for unflavored or lightly flavored types without added sugars or fibers.
- ***Hydrolyzed collagen peptides***: These mix seamlessly into gelatin desserts, supporting not just muscle, but also skin and joint health, especially valuable after substantial weight loss. Note that collagen is not a

complete protein alone ideally, paired with another protein source for full amino acid coverage.

- ***Clear or "ready-to-drink" protein liquid formulations***: Convenient for quickly adding a protein boost to gelatin mixes, these are especially useful if you tire of powders or want a smoother texture.
- ***Approved plant-based protein powders***: With the guidance of your dietitian, pea isolate or rice protein powders may be suitable alternatives for individuals with dairy intolerance.

For flavor, prioritize:

- Sugar-free and alcohol-free flavor extracts (such as vanilla, almond, lemon, or caramel). A few drops are enough to transform a plain gelatin base into a dessert that feels indulgent.
- Bariatric-approved sugar-free syrups for layering or swirling into your finished gelatin for an extra boost in taste.

When integrating any new supplement or extract, check first with your bariatric care team or dietitian for compatibility, dosage, and tolerance.

Sample Recipes Featuring Two or More Complete Protein Sources

Building on this foundation, you can craft gelatin desserts that support your protein quota for the day, stimulate enjoyment of healthy eating, and fit right into your lifelong routine. Below are two sample recipes, each designed to deliver a blend of complete protein sources in a single serving.

Double Protein Delight Gelatin Cup

Ingredients:

- 1 scoop whey isolate (unflavored or vanilla)
- 1 tablespoon hydrolyzed collagen peptides
- 1 packet (calorie-free) unflavored gelatin
- ½ cup unsweetened almond milk (or lactose-free skim milk if tolerated)
- 1 teaspoon sugar-free vanilla extract
- 1–2 teaspoons sugar-free sweetener (stevia or sucralose)

Instructions:

1. In a mixing bowl, bloom the gelatin by sprinkling it over ¼ cup cold milk. Let set 3–5 minutes.
2. Warm the remaining ¼ cup milk in a small saucepan until just steaming, then dissolve the sweetener in it.
3. Pour the hot milk over the bloomed gelatin and stir gently until completely dissolved (do not boil).
4. Whisk in the protein powder and collagen peptides, mixing until smooth (use a blender if needed for uniformity).
5. Stir in the vanilla extract and pour into a ramekin or small glass.
6. Refrigerate for at least 2 hours until set. Enjoy as is, or top with a dab of approved non-fat whipped topping.

Protein-Infused Citrus Gelatin Mousse

Ingredients:

- ½ cup clear, sugar-free lemon or orange gelatin (prepared)
- 1 scoop clear whey protein isolate (citrus-flavored if available)
- 2 tablespoons non-fat Greek yogurt (ensure low lactose)
- 1 teaspoon lemon or orange extract

Instructions:

1. Prepare the sugar-free citrus gelatin as directed, but mix in the protein powder while gelatin is still liquid and slightly warm.
2. Once the gelatin mix cools to room temperature and starts to gel, fold in the Greek yogurt and citrus extract until fully combined and creamy.
3. Pour into a dessert glass and refrigerate until set, at least 2 hours.
4. Serve chilled.

These protein-first gelatin snacks not only meet daily protein quotas but also encourage positive eating behaviors that support long-term success after bariatric surgery.

Sweetener and Topping Compatibility Chart for Protein-First Desserts

Success with gelatin desserts depends as much on safe sweetening and topping options as it does on the protein itself. Bariatric surgery alters your response to sweets; sensitivity is often increased, and consumption of sugar can provoke dumping syndrome or unwanted spikes and crashes in blood sugar. Use this compatibility chart to expand your dessert horizons without sacrificing your health goals.

Approved Sweeteners:

- Stevia (plant-based, non-nutritive)
- Sucralose (found in Splenda and some ready-made gelatins)
- Monkfruit extract
- Erythritol (in moderation, due to potential for GI distress)

Toppings to Use Occasionally (in modest portions, always trialled for tolerance):

- Bariatric-approved non-fat whipped topping
- A dollop of lactose-free Greek yogurt

- Unsweetened pureed fruit (applesauce, peach puree; avoid syrup-packed varieties)
- Grated citrus zest (lemon, lime, or orange)
- Sprinkle of cinnamon or nutmeg

Toppings and Sweeteners to Avoid:

- White or brown sugar, honey, agave, or syrups
- Chocolate chips, candies, or sugared nuts
- Dried fruits or sugary jam/jelly
- Store-bought whipped toppings with added sugar or full fat

Always introduce a new sweetener or topping in a small test batch first, observing for any symptoms of intolerance, excessive sweetness, or triggers for dumping syndrome.

Rules for Fitting Protein Desserts Into Overall Meal Planning Without Risking Dumping Syndrome

Integrating protein-forward gelatin snacks into your eating plan is about much more than satisfying a sweet tooth. To avoid pitfalls like dumping syndrome and hypoglycemia and to prevent protein-rich snacks from crowding out other nutrient needs follow these core principles:

1. ***Prioritize Protein, But Space Out Servings***: Aim for 60 grams of protein per day, spreading it evenly through three main meals and two to three snacks.

Gelatin-based protein desserts should supplement, not replace, your main protein sources.

2. ***Keep Portion Size in Check***: Even protein desserts should be portion-controlled to fit your new stomach size. A typical serving is ½ cup or less. Large or rapid servings of even sugar-free gelatin may cause fullness, nausea, or regurgitation.
3. ***Eat Slowly and Chew Well***: While gelatin is smooth, take small bites and eat slowly. This helps prevent discomfort and supports digestion.
4. ***Never Combine Liquid and Solid Meals***: Wait at least 30 minutes after a meal before consuming a gelatin snack, and do not drink large amounts of fluid at the same time to avoid overfilling your pouch and risking dumping syndrome.
5. ***Avoid Adding Sugars and High-Fat Foods***: Steer clear of hidden sugars and fats that may sneak into toppings or flavorings, as these can trigger dumping syndrome and slow your progress.
6. ***Rotate Flavors and Protein Sources***: This minimizes the chances of palate fatigue and keeps you engaged in your maintenance strategy.
7. ***Monitor Your Body's Response***: Any signs of cramping, bloating, dizziness, or rapid heartbeat suggest the need to adjust recipes, reduce portions, or trial an alternative protein or sweetener.

8. ***Involve Your Care Team***: Continue periodic check-ins with your dietitian, especially when adding new products, making significant changes to your recipe routine, or noticing any negative reactions.When you follow these guidelines and add safe, protein-rich gelatin desserts to your routine, you may help prevent common complications, support optimal nutritional intake, and keep your meals enjoyable over the long term.

Making protein-first gelatin desserts part of your day-to-day eating plan is a sustainable, medically responsible way to support your recovery, muscle mass, and enjoyment of food. With careful selection of protein supplements, flavor extracts, and sweeteners, you can easily rotate several delicious options each week. Most importantly, always align your choices with your own tolerance, medical advice, and nutritional priorities.

When you incorporate protein-enriched gelatin treats into your maintenance phase, you unlock a dessert experience uniquely suited to your needs as a bariatric patient nourishing, satisfying, and fully compatible with your lifelong health journey.

Weekly Meal Plan Featuring Gelatin Snacks and Desserts

A well-structured weekly meal plan is a cornerstone for recovery and long-term maintenance after bariatric surgery. When it comes to gelatin snacks and desserts, thoughtful planning supports consistent protein intake, helps manage hydration, and lessens the stress of day-to-day food preparation.

This chapter provides you with a realistic, medically responsible weekly meal schedule, practical batch prep strategies, and concrete tools for tracking your intake ensuring that your gelatin treats are always safe, stage-appropriate, and enjoyable as you recover.

Seven-Day Sample Gelatin Snack/Dessert Schedule Aligned With Bariatric Eating Times

To maximize your nutrition and uphold healthy eating behavior after bariatric surgery, it's recommended to eat small, frequent meals and snacks, typically every 2–4 hours during waking hours. Because the volume your stomach can hold is much smaller, meeting your protein and hydration goals takes strategic timing especially in the early stages of post-operative care when your ability to eat solids is limited and texture progression is gradual.

Below is a seven-day gelatin snack schedule that fits typical bariatric post-surgery eating times, aligning with each diet progression stage. Adjustments should always reflect your individual advancement and medical advice.

Day 1–2: Clear Liquid Stage

- ***Mid-morning***: 1–2 oz (30–60 ml) protein-fortified, sugar-free clear gelatin (e.g., lemon flavor, made with unflavored clear whey protein isolate)
- ***Mid-afternoon***: 1–2 oz (30–60 ml) sugar-free gelatin (no added cream or puree ingredients)
- ***Evening***: 1 oz (30 ml) clear gelatin cube for hydration and light snacking

Day 3–4: Full Liquid Stage

- ***Mid-morning***: 2 oz (60 ml) protein-enhanced gelatin mousse (prepared with non-fat dairy or non-dairy alternatives as tolerated)
- ***Afternoon***: 2 oz (60 ml) sugar-free berry gelatin cup with added clear protein supplement
- ***Early evening***: 1–2 oz (30–60 ml) vanilla-pudding style gelatin

Day 5–7: Transition to Pureed/Soft Stage

- ***Morning***: 2–3 oz (60–90 ml) soft-set gelatin blended with approved pureed fruit or non-fat Greek yogurt
- ***Afternoon***: 2 oz (60 ml) protein-first gelatin parfait, layered with whipped, sugar-free topping
- ***Evening***: 1–2 oz (30–60 ml) soft 'fluff' gelatin (whipped for light texture), flavored with citrus or vanilla extract

Regular Maintenance Phase (Sample Snack Slots for an Ongoing Week)

1. Monday/Wednesday/Friday
   - Mid-morning: ½ cup (120 ml) high-protein gelatin dessert (whey or pea protein plus gelatin, sugar-free flavor)
   - Afternoon: ½ cup (120 ml) protein-enhanced gelatin mousse, rotating flavors to prevent palate fatigue

2. Tuesday/Thursday/Saturday
   - Noon: ½ cup (120 ml) berry-citrus sugar-free gelatin, layered with 2 Tbsp lactose-free Greek yogurt (if tolerated)
   - Evening: ¼–½ cup (60–120 ml) tropical protein gelatin snack (pineapple extract, unflavored protein supplement)

3. Sunday

- Snack: ½ cup (120 ml) "double protein" gelatin cup (mixture of collagen peptides and clear whey protein)
- Optional: 2–3 gelatin "cubes" (approx. 1 oz/30 ml each) for evening hydration

This schedule is meant to supplement not replace your regular small meals, which remain focused around high-quality protein and produce. Always advance texture or portion only after demonstrating tolerance at your current stage and with the approval of your bariatric team.

Portion Size Cheat Sheet Matching Stage-Appropriate Intake Volumes

Portion control is central to both comfort and safety after surgery. The following cheat sheet summarizes guideline portion sizes for gelatin snacks through each diet phase. These sizes help prevent regurgitation, minimize fullness or discomfort, and support safe progression:

Clear Liquid:

1–2 oz (30–60 ml) per snack, sipped or taken in small, slow spoonfuls

Full Liquid:

2 oz (60 ml) per serving, up to twice per day

Pureed/Soft:

2–3 oz (60–90 ml) per snack, with smooth or blended additions as tolerated

Regular/Long-term Maintenance:

¼–½ cup (60–120 ml) per snack/dessert, eaten slowly (over 10–15 minutes)

Always remember to eat smaller amounts if you experience fullness or discomfort.

Chew thoroughly, especially if adding soft fruits, eat slowly, and continue to avoid drinking liquids during meals, as current guidelines for post-bariatric patients still recommend against consuming fluids with food.

Overconsumption of gelatin may potentially cause nausea, bloating, or discomfort, particularly in individuals with a reduced gastric pouch size; however, this effect has not been widely documented in clinical guidelines or studies.

Batch Preparation Worksheet for Efficient, Safe Weekly Gelatin Cooking

Saving time and ensuring food safety is easier with batch preparation. Here is an efficient worksheet to guide your weekly gelatin snack prep:

1. **Calculate Your Weekly Needs:**
    - How many snacks do you need per week? (Usually 7–14, depending on your eating pattern and stage)
    - What stage-appropriate serving sizes are you preparing? (Refer to the cheat sheet above)

2. **Choose Flavors and Protein Types:**
    - Pick 2–3 sugar-free gelatin flavors (rotate to prevent palate fatigue)
    - Decide on protein additions: unflavored whey isolate, clear protein liquid, or hydrolyzed collagen (as approved)
    - Select any Stage 3+ add-ins (pureed fruit, yogurt)

3. **Prepare Your Gelatin Recipe Base:**
    - Follow exact temperature rules: Never add protein powder to water hotter than 140°F (60°C) this prevents clumping and nutrient loss
    - Mix sweetener and protein with liquid before blooming gelatin, then warm gently to dissolve, stir until completely smooth

4. **Portion and Chill:**
    - Pour prepared gelatin into stage-appropriate pre-measured containers (e.g., 2 oz/60 ml reusable cups for early stages; ½ cup/120 ml ramekins for maintenance)

- Cover containers and refrigerate immediately on the upper fridge shelf (never at room temperature)

5. **Label and Date:**

   Label each portion with flavor, add-ins, date of preparation, and "use by" deadline (usually 3–5 days for freshly made gelatin, if kept refrigerated and covered)

6. **Store Safely:**
   - Keep gelatin away from raw food
   - Always wash hands, utensils, and preparation surfaces thoroughly to prevent contamination

7. **Rotate Batches:**

   Use "first in, first out" principle to avoid old portions lingering in your fridge

This worksheet helps you efficiently plan and batch-cook without exceeding your food safety comfort zone or intake limits.

Food Log Template for Tracking Protein, Calories, and Hydration From Gelatin Foods

Systematic food tracking reinforces your success by making nutrient intake and hydration measurable. Use this simple, bariatric-specific food log for gelatin-based snacks and desserts throughout each week:

Table 4: Food Log Entry Example

Date	Snack Time	Recipe Name/ Flavor	Portion Size (oz/ml)	Protein (g)	Calories	Fluid Contribution (ml)	Notes/ Tolerance
6/1	10:00 AM	Lemon Whey Gelatin	2 oz (60)	12	45	55	No discomfort
6/1	2:30 PM	Berry Gel Mousse	2 oz (60)	10	50	50	Felt a little full—eat slower next time

Tips for maximizing your food log:

- Record each gelatin snack promptly after eating to avoid forgetfulness
- Note any symptoms (bloating, fullness, taste aversion, etc.) and share during care visits
- Track your total daily protein from all sources to ensure you meet or exceed the 60 g/day minimum (or your team's individualized goal)
- Don't forget to include the fluid volume from gelatin snacks in your total daily hydration calculations

When used consistently, this log helps adjust recipes, portion sizes, or protein concentrations as your needs change and gives your care team valuable data for future recommendations.

Sample Shopping List for a Week of Bariatric-Friendly Gelatin Ingredients

Filling your kitchen with the right supplies ensures you're always ready to whip up protein-focused, sugar-free treats that honor both your tastes and medical guidelines. Here's a model shopping list for a week of gelatin-based snacks and desserts (adjust amounts according to household size and weekly batch):

Essential Ingredients:

- Sugar-free flavored gelatin mix (3–4 different flavors, as tolerated; look for those sweetened with sucralose, stevia, or aspartame)
- Unflavored gelatin packets (for custom flavors or use with clear protein drinks)
- Clear whey protein isolate or hydrolyzed collagen peptides (check with dietitian for brand recommendations)
- Sugar-free flavor extracts (vanilla, lemon, almond, orange, etc.)
- Non-fat Greek yogurt (lactose-free, low sugar; for Stage 3 and above)
- Sugar-free non-dairy or dairy milk (unsweetened almond, lactose-free skim, etc.)
- Stevia or monkfruit extract (granular or liquid for homemade sweetening)

- Bariatric-approved clear protein liquid supplements (ready-made or concentrate, for easy mixing)
- Fresh lemon or lime (for zest or juice in custom gelatin blends)

Optional Stage-3+ Items:

- Approved pureed fruit (unsweetened, low fiber; such as applesauce or peach puree)
- Bariatric-approved non-fat whipped topping (check ingredient label for no sugar or full fat)

Supplies:

- Reusable portion cups (2 oz/60 ml and ½ cup/120 ml sizes)
- Ramekins or glass dessert dishes with lids
- Food-safe labels and marker
- Mixing bowl, whisk, and spatula

Shopping tips:

- Verify product labels for sugar content, artificial sweetener types, and protein per serving—avoid hidden sugars or excess fat
- Buy in quantities scaled to your batch-prep plan to avoid waste and ensure safety

Keeping your kitchen stocked with these essentials, you'll be able to prepare snacks that meet your protein and hydration needs, satisfy your sweet tooth, and respect your post-surgical limitations. This proactive approach will also help you avoid last-minute purchases of items that might not meet your medical criteria or portion guidelines.

Key Reminders for Success

- Refer to your individual post-op diet stage and consult with your bariatric dietitian before introducing new flavors, proteins, or add-ins
- Space out snacks from meals and accompany each with mindful, slow eating to support optimal digestion and nutrient absorption
- Monitor for any signs of food intolerance, allergic reaction, or dumping syndrome, and log these in your food diary for reference
- Hydration is as critical as protein count the liquid component of gelatin snacks toward your daily fluid intake, but do not substitute gelatin for all fluid needs

A methodical, stage-appropriate gelatin snack plan does more than make recovery easier—it empowers you with flexibility, flavor variety, and confidence in meeting protein and hydration requirements during every week of your bariatric journey.

Implement this plan and tailor it to your personal preferences, digestion, and lifestyle to ensure that high-protein gelatin snacks remain a sustainable, enjoyable, and effective part of your recovery and lifelong maintenance.

Safe Storage, Handling, and Food Safety for Homemade Gelatin

Proper storage and handling of homemade gelatin are essential for bariatric patients, as food safety plays a crucial role in recovery, appetite, and nutrient preservation. Because post-surgical eating volume is small, snacks are often made in batches, stored for several days, and eaten slowly.

Missteps in food handling or storage can increase your risk for foodborne illness, compromise the delicate protein blends in bariatric-friendly gelatin, or even lead to inadvertent dietary setbacks. This chapter distills expert best practices for keeping your homemade gelatin snacks safe, appealing, and appropriately nutritious at every stage of your bariatric journey.

Recommended storage containers and cooling times to maintain food safety and texture

Choosing the right storage containers for gelatin is not just about convenience—it protects both food quality and your health. Immediately after preparing gelatin, portion it into single-serve containers that align with your program's recommended serving sizes: for example, many standard bariatric recovery guidelines suggest using 2 oz (60 ml) cups for early postoperative stages, and ½ cup (120 ml) or similar ramekins for later or maintenance stages.

Always confirm portion sizes with your healthcare provider or refer to your specific program's standards. These individual-size containers reduce risk of cross-contamination and help control serving sizes, thus lowering the chance of overeating or introduction of too-solid food textures too soon.

Select containers that are:

- BPA-free and food-safe (plastic, glass, or silicone)
- Airtight with a secure lid to prevent moisture loss or absorption of fridge odors
- Opaque or semi-transparent when possible, as exposure to light and air can alter flavors and degrade sensitive nutrients found in protein-fortified gelatin

For optimal texture and sanitation, pour gelatin mixtures into portioned containers while still liquid, cover immediately, and allow them to cool on the kitchen counter just until "steam" disappears (no more than 30 minutes). Then, promptly transfer them to the upper shelf of the refrigerator where the temperature is most stable and coldest, ideally 4°C (39°F) or slightly below.

Never leave homemade gelatin unrefrigerated for more than one hour, as the protein content and low-acid environment can support bacterial growth. Quick cooling also ensures a smooth gel set, preventing graininess or separation common if the mixture remains at room temperature too long.

Gelatin batch storage timeframes for each stage with discard rule chart

Each post-bariatric diet stage comes with its own demands from smaller, more frequent snacks to the need for gradual texture progression. Below is a simple chart summarizing how long you can safely keep homemade gelatin for each stage and when to discard any leftovers:

Table 5: Discard Rule Chart

Diet Stage	Storage Time (Refrigerated)	Discard/Use By Rule
Clear/Full Liquid (Stage 1/2)	Up to 3 days	Discard if not used within 72 hours
Pureed/Soft (Stage 3/4)	Up to 4 days	Discard after 96 hours from prep time
Maintenance (Regular)	Up to 5 days	Discard after 120 hours

Regardless of the stage, if at any point a gelatin snack shows any signs of spoilage (such as off-smell, visible mold, separation, or flavor change), it should be discarded immediately even if it is within the suggested storage window.

Always use the "first in, first out" method: place newly prepared batches of snacks behind older ones in your fridge so that the oldest snacks are eaten first, reducing the risk of spoilage. This is especially important after bariatric surgery, as maintaining food safety is crucial for your recovery and health.

Storage and reheating checklist to avoid contamination and nutrient degradation

Maintaining safety and nutritional value in your homemade gelatin starts before storage and continues until you take the first bite. Here's a focused checklist for optimal results:

- Wash hands thoroughly before and after preparing gelatin and before touching containers or utensils at any time this is especially important for post-bariatric patients who may have a temporarily compromised immune status.
- Sanitize work surfaces, mixing bowls, whisks, and all utensils before use and between batch preps, especially if preparing varieties with dairy, fruit, or unflavored protein additions.
- Use only clean, dry containers with tight lids for storage.
- Chill gelatin quickly: place briefly on the counter, cover, and then refrigerate immediately. Do not allow

warm gelatin to sit at room temperature, as bacteria multiply fastest when foods are cooled slowly.

- Store on top shelves, away from raw meat, fish, or eggs to avoid cross-contamination.
- Avoid stacking gelatin containers directly on top of each other when first cooling; leave space for cold air to circulate.
- Never reheat gelatin. Unlike hearty soups or stews, gelatin snacks should always be eaten cold or at fridge temperature. Reheating can break down the protein network, destroy added nutrients, and encourage bacteria growth if the snack is held too long in the "danger zone" temperature range. If a snack becomes too firm, rest it at room temperature for just 5–10 minutes before eating (but always return uneaten portions to the fridge quickly).

Labeling and portioning techniques for managing multiple snack types in the fridge

It is common to have several snack varieties with different flavors, protein concentrations, or recipes for household members at different recovery stages in your fridge at once. Clear labeling prevents confusion, ensures everyone's safety, and supports adherence to your plan.

Effective labeling and portioning strategies include:

- Use food-grade, removable labels with space for date of preparation, flavor/protein type, stage-appropriateness, and use-by date.
- Color-code lids or containers if preparing for multiple people or stages for example, blue for clear liquid, green for full liquid, orange for pureed/soft, and red for maintenance.
- Write serving size in large print on each container, so you never confuse a Stage 1 snack with a regular-sized dessert.
- Store similar snack types together in designated fridge "zones" or a dedicated plastic bin, so you can quickly find today's approved snack without rummaging through the fridge.
- When batch prepping, portion out gelatin using pre-measured cups/spoons to avoid the temptation of "fudging" serving sizes, which can undermine your progress or lead to accidental overconsumption.

Labeling isn't just for organization, it is part of food safety. Knowing exactly when each container was prepped and when it should be used up prevents accidental consumption of out-of-date snacks and supports consistency in your nutrient tracking efforts.

Signs of spoilage or poor storage outcomes and corrective steps

Consuming spoiled or mishandled food can jeopardize recovery, trigger gastrointestinal upset, or, in serious cases, lead to foodborne illness risks heightened during the immunologically-suppressed post-surgical period. As gelatin is a high-moisture, protein-enriched food, it is important to recognize when a batch may be unsafe.

Common signs your homemade gelatin should be discarded immediately:

- Any visible mold, even a small spot
- A sour, yeasty, or off-putting odor upon opening the container
- Unusual separation of liquid at the base or on surface (especially if milky or cloudy)
- Surface texture appears slimy, sticky, or if the gel no longer holds its set shape
- Change in color or presence of "bubbles" not seen when first prepared
- Any odd flavor on first bite do not continue eating to "test it out"

If you notice any of the above, throw out the entire container, do not attempt to scrape off the top or "cut away" suspicious areas, as bacteria and mold penetrate below the visible surface.

Corrective steps to avoid spoilage in the future include:

- Ensuring that gelatin mixes and protein powders are fresh, properly sealed between uses, and not used past their expiration date
- Maintaining a consistent, cold fridge temperature (4°C or 39°F)
- Avoiding preparation of more snacks than you can reasonably consume within the safe storage window for your current diet stage
- Keeping prepared gelatin well-covered at all times, even while serving, to prevent airborne contamination
- Strictly adhering to your discard/use-by chart; when in doubt, always err on the side of caution

Remember that certain symptoms experienced after eating spoiled gelatin may mimic early dumping or intolerance (nausea, bloating, abdominal discomfort), but spoilage poses additional health risks. If in doubt about your symptoms or snack safety, consult your bariatric care team promptly.

Final Safety Reminders for Bariatric Gelatin Success

Following these storage and handling practices protects the investment you make in each safe, protein-focused gelatin batch and minimizes setbacks in your bariatric recovery. Food safety is as fundamental as recipe selection or portion control, and no stage of post-op eating can succeed without it. Here are your final reminders:

- Always wash hands and sanitize workspaces before and during all food prep
- Label every single container with critical information ditch any "mystery snack" in your fridge
- Store gelatin promptly, at the right temperature, and keep covered at all times
- Eat snacks within their specified safe window never risk eating anything questionable, no matter how well it seems to "smell" or "look"
- Never reheat gelatin snacks; always consume cold or at fridge temperature
- Regularly review your fridge's contents, rotating new batches to the back and moving older ones forward

When you incorporate these routines into your weekly snack preparation, you help ensure that each homemade gelatin treat supports, rather than jeopardizes, your post-bariatric recovery. Safe storage and careful handling offer confidence to enjoy the flexibility and flavor of gelatin snacks throughout each stage of your diet. This approach maximizes the benefits of your bariatric surgery investment and helps maintain consistency in your nutritional journey.

Troubleshooting Common Problems With Bariatric Gelatin Recipes

Creating bariatric gelatin snacks after surgery is not just about following a recipe, it's about meeting your texture tolerance, nutrient, and flavor needs as you recover. While gelatin recipes are valuable tools for providing hydration and protein during your staged diet, challenges may crop up along the way.

Whether you're dealing with digestive side effects, experiencing flavor fatigue, puzzling over a batch that won't set quite right, or facing the consequences of advancing textures too rapidly, knowing how to troubleshoot common problems allows you to stay safe, comfortable, and compliant with your nutrition plan.

This chapter offers structured checklists, simple fixes, and clear communication strategies so you can confidently address barriers and keep your recovery on track.

Digestive Side Effect Identification Checklist: Intolerance, Nausea, and Sweetener Issues

The first signal that a gelatin snack isn't working for you is how you feel after eating it. Because the post-bariatric digestive tract is more sensitive due to anatomical and hormonal changes, it's common to experience side effects if a snack is too sweet, too large, or contains problematic ingredients.

Use the following checklist to quickly evaluate your reaction to a new gelatin recipe:

- Nausea or queasiness within minutes to half an hour of eating
- Bloating, gassiness, or abdominal discomfort
- Unusual fullness or regurgitation after even small servings
- Loose stools, diarrhea, or increased trips to the bathroom
- Sweetness "burn" an unpleasant aftertaste or overwhelming flavor, especially from artificial sweeteners
- Lightheadedness, palpitations, or sweating possible early dumping symptoms if the gelatin is not truly sugar-free, or contains hidden rapidly-absorbed carbohydrates

- Fatigue, shakiness, or confusion appearing 1–3 hours after a snack could indicate late dumping or reactive hypoglycemia

These symptoms overlap with both food intolerance and complications such as dumping syndrome or postprandial hypoglycemia, which are more likely to occur post-surgery. Since bariatric surgery increases sensitivity to sweet tastes and changes how your body reacts to certain foods, even a small recipe tweak like a new protein blend or sweetener can trigger discomfort.

If you identify one or more of the above symptoms after trying a gelatin recipe:

- Stop eating the snack immediately.
- Track what you ate, how much, and when the symptoms appeared.
- Review ingredient labels for hidden sugars or non-approved sweeteners.
- Note if new supplements or protein powders were just introduced.

These records help you and your care team pinpoint problem foods and prevent repeat episodes.

Flavor Fatigue Signals and Rotation Tactics for Maintaining Interest and Compliance

With medical restrictions narrowing ingredient options, eating the same gelatin snack day after day often leads to "flavor fatigue," a major threat to long-term compliance and nutrition intake. Recognizing when boredom is setting in is crucial:

- Less interest in eating snacks you once enjoyed
- Skipping gelatin servings or feeling "repulsed" by a previously favored flavor
- Reaching for non-compliant foods out of a desire for a different taste or texture
- Reporting "nothing tastes good anymore"

After bariatric surgery, your palate and hedonic appreciation of sweets and fatty foods are altered—not only are you more sensitive to sweet flavors, but your body may actively develop subtle aversions if a specific taste or food frequently causes gastrointestinal discomfort.

This adaptation, called conditioned taste avoidance, can shift over time and is intensified if a particular recipe leads to nausea, bloating, or fullness repeatedly. In practice, this means flavor rotation isn't just about staving off boredom, but also about keeping your snacks tolerable and stimulating your appetite.

Rotation tactics include:

- Prepare small batches using two to three different flavors each week, rather than one large batch of a single variety.
- Alternate between citrus, berry, and "creamy" flavor profiles if permitted by your stage.
- Try rotating types of protein supplement added to gelatin (whey isolate vs. collagen peptides) for subtle changes in taste and mouthfeel.
- Incorporate allowed flavor extracts (such as vanilla, almond, lemon, or coconut) in varying proportions.
- Use different serving vessels, small molds, ramekins, or "mini cubes" to change perceived texture or presentation.

Staying attentive to flavor fatigue signals and being proactive with rotation will support long-term adherence and make gelatin recipes a sustainable part of your bariatric toolkit. Remember that some early sensitivity to sweetness or aroma is normal while your palate recalibrates; if you're unsure whether fatigue is physical or psychological, document when the shift began and discuss with your care team.

Texture Troubleshooting Guide for Fixes (Too Runny, Grainy, or Dense Gel Results)

A major benefit of homemade bariatric gelatin is the ability to control texture crucial as your diet advances from clear liquids to regular foods. However, some batches may not set or blend as planned. Common texture complaints and solutions include:

Too Runny (Fails to Set)

- Likely Cause: Insufficient gelatin concentration, excess fluid, or poor mixing.
- Fix: Double-check gelatin-to-liquid ratios. For protein-enriched recipes, dissolve protein powders completely before mixing with gelatin base to prevent dilution.
- If using unflavored collagen or protein, bloom (soften) the gelatin in a small amount of liquid first, then mix into warm, not boiling liquids and allow full chilling time in the fridge.

Grainy or Lumpy

- Likely Cause: Inefficient protein powder dispersion or overheating.
- Fix: Sift protein powder before whisking into the liquid; mix thoroughly while liquids are warm but not hot.
- Avoid boiling liquids when mixing with gelatin, as high heat denatures proteins leading to curdled or grainy texture.
- Use immersion blenders for best smoothness if adding dense powders.

Too Firm or Dense

- Likely Cause: Excess gelatin or inadequate liquid, especially when adding high-protein supplements.
- Fix: Reduce the gelatin powder slightly, or increase the approved liquid (water, broth, or permitted milk substitute) in the recipe.
- If already set, try blending the gel with a small amount of extra liquid and resetting individual portions.

Protein-enriched gelatins are more sensitive to proportion and mixing technique due to the structure of added proteins, so precise measurement and gentle, thorough mixing are key. If every batch has texture issues, adjust your preparation technique before altering the recipe, sometimes simply allowing mixtures to rest, thoroughly dissolving all powders, or making smaller batches can correct persistent problems.

Action Plan for When Solid Foods Are Accidentally Introduced Too Soon Via Gelatin Snacks

Diet progression after bariatric surgery is deliberately staged to protect your healing stomach and intestines. Accidentally adding solid elements (such as fruit chunks, seeds, or chewy inclusions) to gelatin snacks ahead of schedule can introduce complications, including regurgitation, vomiting, or even physical discomfort.

If you realize that a snack with solid components was consumed before your care team has approved advancement:

1. Stop eating the snack immediately.
2. Do not attempt to "solve" the issue by consuming more food or fluid, which could worsen symptoms.
3. Monitor for regurgitation, nausea, vomiting, abdominal pain, and early symptoms of dumping syndrome.
4. If symptoms are mild (light nausea or discomfort), rest and sip only clear approved fluids in small sips for 30–60 minutes.
5. For ongoing or worsening symptoms, contact your bariatric team for instructions especially if vomiting, persistent pain, or signs of obstruction develop.

Generally, most protocols recommend a liquid or very soft diet in the first days post-op, with gradual progression in texture over several weeks; introducing too-solid food can destabilize your recovery or slow adaptation to your new anatomy. Always carefully check recipes and ingredients and, if prepping for multiple people or stages, label containers to eliminate accidental introduction of advanced textures.

If you accidentally ate a denser gelatin snack, use the following caution plan until cleared by your team:

- Avoid all solids for at least 24 hours.
- Increase the frequency of very small, clear liquid intakes.

- Document the incident: what, when, how much, symptoms experienced.
- Contact your bariatric team if any concerning symptoms appear.

Communication Template for Reporting and Documenting Issues to Your Bariatric Care Team

When digestive or compliance problems arise even with carefully prepared gelatin snacks, clear, structured communication with your bariatric team is vital for safety and effective recovery planning. Reporting not just what happened, but also the specific product and your timing with respect to your surgical phase, allows your care team to give detailed, informed guidance.

<u>*Use this template to prepare for calls, emails, or appointments:*</u>

<u>***Subject: Bariatric Gelatin Snack Reaction/Problem Report***</u>

Patient Name:

Surgery Type and Date:

Current Diet Stage:

Date/Time of Problem Snack:

Gelatin Recipe or Product Used:

- Brand and flavor (if commercial) or recipe/protein/sweetener used (if homemade)
- Portion size and time consumed

Description of Reaction:

- Onset and duration of symptoms (nausea, bloating, palpitations, diarrhea, etc.)
- Severity (mild, moderate, severe; able/unable to continue normal activities)
- Was any solid or unapproved food introduced (intentionally or by mistake)?

Actions Taken:

- Stopped eating, fluids taken, rest, medications used
- Change in hydration, appetite, or other foods since the reaction

Questions/Concerns:

- Need for next steps in management?
- Dietary adjustments or ingredient changes recommended?
- Future risk or long-term consequences to watch for?

Collaborating with your care team using this structured information supports accurate assessment, focused advice, and appropriate changes to your nutrition plan. It also arms you with the confidence to advocate for your comfort and safety as you experiment with new recipes or adjust your snack routines.

Troubleshooting challenges with bariatric gelatin recipes is a normal part of adapting to post-surgical nutrition. By recognizing and responding to digestive side effects, rotating flavors to prevent fatigue, fine-tuning batch textures, and communicating clearly with your care team, you turn small setbacks into important learning moments. The result: more comfortable enjoyment of protein-rich, sugar-free gelatin snacks that truly work for your unique stage and situation. As you progress, keep this guide handy, experiment thoughtfully, respect your body's signals, and reach out for help whenever a hurdle arises. Consistent troubleshooting ensures gelatin snacks remain a safe, appealing, and sustainable part of your long-term bariatric nutritional strategy.

Conclusion

Sustaining success with bariatric gelatin snacks requires ongoing attention to nutrition, texture, and behavioral habits as you navigate each stage of recovery and establish new long-term routines. Gelatin-based treats are not just a temporary fix when selected and prepared well, they can be a flavorful, reliable component of your protein-first, sugar-free diet for months and years after surgery.

A key strategy for ongoing success is to remain vigilant about your protein intake. Maintaining protein intake above 60 grams per day is recommended for most post-bariatric patients, as it helps minimize the loss of fat-free and muscle mass during the rapid weight loss phase. Because reaching this target with natural foods alone is often difficult in the early months, especially when appetite or tolerance is low, protein-enriched gelatin snacks offer a practical means to boost your intake without overwhelming your restricted stomach capacity. As your recovery progresses, continue to monitor your total protein across all meals, integrating protein-first gelatin treats as a routine snack or dessert to help meet your needs.

Behavioral follow-through is just as important as recipe selection. Research shows that patients who receive structured dietary counseling and incorporate behavioral strategies to support their new eating patterns experience greater weight loss and long-term compliance. Consider establishing rituals around your snack preparation batch-making gelatin desserts at set times each week, portioning them into labeled containers, and tracking your intake with a simple food and hydration log. If you notice lapses in your routines or start skipping snack servings, return to your checklist and discuss any emerging challenges with your care team.

To maintain flavor variety and palatability, keep rotating gelatin flavors and protein add-ins. This not only prevents taste fatigue but also supports appetite and minimizes the risk of developing food aversions, a phenomenon that is common after bariatric surgery due to the interplay of altered gut hormones and learned taste avoidance when certain foods cause post-meal discomfort. A flexible, rotating approach also allows you to adapt recipes when ingredient availability or personal preferences shift over time, all while staying within stage-appropriate guidelines.

Cautiously advancing texture and volume is essential as you move from the liquid to the regular diet phase. Always adhere to your bariatric center's progression protocol, which relies on the principle of gradually increasing food consistency to avoid regurgitation or vomiting in the early post-op period. When introducing new or denser gelatin snacks, such as parfaits or mousse blends, start with very small portions and increase only after confirming tolerance. If in doubt, consult with your dietary team before trying a more advanced recipe.

Regularly reassessing your overall dietary strategy is also critical. Continued nutritional counseling, at least in the first year after surgery, can protect against setbacks and reinforce positive behaviors. Should protein intake, texture tolerance, or flavor acceptance become problematic, do not hesitate to reach out for professional guidance early intervention can prevent minor issues from deterring your recovery.

Finally, keep safety top of mind by following strict food handling, storage, and batch preparation protocols. Labeling, proper chilling, and observing recommended discard timeframes not only maintain the integrity of your snacks but also reduce the risk of digestive complications, which can be heightened by improper food safety post-surgery.

In summary, the foundation for ongoing bariatric gelatin success is a blend of practical preparation habits, diligent protein monitoring, behavioral reinforcement, flavor and texture flexibility, and close partnership with your care team. Incorporating these strategies will support not just your recovery, but also enjoyable, sustainable eating well into your new, healthier life.

FAQs

Can gelatin snacks replace other protein supplements during early recovery stages?

Gelatin snacks can be a useful addition to your early post-bariatric diet, but they should not replace traditional protein supplements in the critical first months after surgery. Achieving adequate protein intake at least 60 grams per day, or up to 1.5 grams per kilogram of ideal body weight is vital for healing. Since eating enough solid, protein-rich foods is difficult right after surgery, liquid protein supplements (usually providing 30 grams per day) are typically recommended.

Gelatin snacks, especially those fortified with protein powders or protein drinks, can help you reach your protein goals and provide hydration, but plain gelatin is low in protein and lacks a complete amino acid profile. For best results, use protein-fortified gelatin snacks as a supplement to not a replacement for formulated protein supplements until you can tolerate solid protein foods.

What artificial sweeteners are best tolerated by post-bariatric patients in gelatin recipes?

After bariatric surgery, taste preferences and sensitivity to sweetness often change, and some sweeteners can trigger symptoms like dumping syndrome. The most tolerated options in gelatin recipes are non-nutritive sweeteners that don't cause rapid sugar absorption or digestive upset, such as sucralose, stevia, and acesulfame potassium.

These don't spike blood sugar or typically cause dumping. Avoid sugar alcohols like sorbitol and maltitol if you're prone to bloating or diarrhea, and always check product labels for hidden sugars. Try new sweeteners gradually and monitor for discomfort, adjusting recipes as needed.

How should I adapt gelatin snacks if I have lactose intolerance?

Lactose intolerance is common after bariatric surgery. To adapt gelatin snacks, avoid milk, cream, yogurt, or lactose-containing protein powders. Use water, broth, lactose-free milk, unsweetened plant-based milks, or clear, lactose-free protein drinks instead.

If you want to boost protein content, choose protein isolate powders labeled lactose-free (like whey isolate, pea, or soy). For creamier snacks, unsweetened soy or almond milk can be used if tolerated. Since gelatin itself is lactose-free, stick with unflavored gelatin and safe, lactose-free flavorings to minimize risk.

What signs indicate a gelatin snack is causing dumping syndrome or similar problems?

Dumping syndrome can happen after bariatric surgery, especially with Roux-en-Y gastric bypass or sleeve gastrectomy, and is triggered by foods high in sugar or rapidly absorbed carbs. Early dumping (within 15 minutes) may cause heart palpitations, flushing, nausea, diarrhea, or bloating.

Late dumping (1–3 hours later) can cause shakiness, sweating, weakness, confusion, or intense hunger. If you notice these symptoms after eating gelatin snacks, the recipe may be too high in sugar or sweeteners, or you may be eating too much too quickly. Smaller, more frequent snacks and delayed fluid intake (waiting 30 minutes after eating before drinking) can help reduce risk.

How can I add more protein to homemade gelatin without impacting texture or flavor?

To increase protein, dissolve unflavored protein isolate (like whey, collagen, or soy) in a small amount of cool water before mixing it into warm, dissolved gelatin. For a creamier result, add unsweetened plant milk or lactose-free alternatives as your diet allows. Avoid boiling protein powders to prevent an unpleasant texture. Start with small amounts and adjust as tolerated. If the texture is too dense, reduce gelatin or increase liquid slightly.

Is it safe to prepare gelatin snacks in advance and freeze them?

You can safely refrigerate gelatin snacks in single portions for up to 3–5 days. Freezing is technically safe, but often changes the texture, making snacks watery or rubbery after thawing. Test a single portion before freezing larger batches. Always label and date containers, and discard any with off odors, excess moisture, or mold.

How often should I check in with my care team about new gelatin recipes or snack changes?

Regular contact with your bariatric care team is important, especially when trying new foods or recipes. Discuss new ingredients or snacks with your surgeon or dietitian during each follow-up, or sooner if you notice intolerance, difficulty meeting protein/hydration goals, or want to change your diet stage. Keep a food and symptom log to share at appointments. Prompt communication helps prevent setbacks and supports steady recovery.

References and Helpful Links

Kelly, P. Whey protein ingredient applications. In Whey proteins (pp. 335-375). Academic Press. 2019. https://doi.org/10.1016/B978-0-12-812124-5.00010-2

Middleton, K. R., Anton, S. D., & Perri, M. G. (2013). Long-term adherence to health behavior change. American journal of lifestyle medicine, 7(6), 395-404. 2013. https://journals.sagepub.com/doi/abs/10.1177/1559827613488867

Parkes, E. Nutritional Management of Patients after Bariatric Surgery. The American Journal of the Medical Sciences. doi:10./-0-7. 20. https://www.sciencedirect.com/science/article/pii/S0002962915328081

MACHELLA, T. THE MECHANISM OF THE POST-GASTRECTOMY "DUMPING" SYNDROME. Annals of Surgery. doi:10./-0-1. 19. https://journals.lww.com/annalsofsurgery/citation/1949/08000/The_Mechanism_of_the_Post_Gastrectomy__Dumping_.1.aspx

Van Der Rest, M. Garrone, R.. Collagen family of proteins. The FASEB Journal. doi:10./fasebj.5.13.105. 19. https://faseb.onlinelibrary.wiley.com/doi/abs/10.1096/fasebj.5.13.1916105

Cincione, R. Losavio, F., Cibelli, G. et al.. Revised Protein Sparing Diet in Obesity and Type 2 Diabetes Mellitus. Nutrients. doi:10./nu. 20. https://www.mdpi.com/2072-6643/14/24/5325

Damodaran, S., Paraf, A.. Food Proteins and their Applications. https://doi.org/10.1201/9780203755617

Schubert, J. Csordas, A.. Imaging of the Gastrointestinal Tract and Bariatric Surgery. Bariatric Surgery. doi:10./7-27. 20. n.d.. https://www.taylorfrancis.com/chapters/edit/10.1201/9781003522737-27/imaging-gastrointestinal-tract-bariatric-surgery-johanna-schubert-attila-csordas

Oniang'o, R.. Food Safety. https://doi.org/10.18697/ajfand119.ed128

www.ingramcontent.com/pod-product-compliance
Lightning Source LLC
LaVergne TN
LVHW022005200926
848481LV00007B/2240